Outcome Standards in Home Health:

State of the Art

Lynn T. Rinke, MS, RN

Pub. No. 21-2204

National League for Nursing • New York

CONTENTS

INTRODUCTION

Just as cost containment has driven health policy decision making in the 70s and 80s, quality has quickly become the focus of health policy for the late 80s and 90s. But in an era of cost consciousness and increasing accountability, claiming to deliver quality health care is not enough. The purchasers of health care -- the government, business, individual consumers -- want to know what their dollar is buying. In the increasingly diversified health care marketplace, new and more precise ways of determining quality are being sought. The central issue is how to judge the quality of the outcome of the delivered health care. Indeed, health policymakers concur that the time has come to identify and quantify the outcomes of the health care system.

The simplest health care outcome to identify and measure is mortality. In fact the Health Care Financing Administration (HCFA), over strident opposition from the American Medical Association (AMA) and the American Hospital Association (AHA), recently "bit the bullet" and made a policy decision to release mortality data to the public. Many hospital spokespeople have gone to great lengths to explain why the data is not intrepretable. Explanations attempt to demonstrate that a particular hospital's patients are different than those of neighboring hospitals: the patients are older, sicker, poorer, have a greater number of co-morbidities, and so forth. Some hospital however are clearly citing mortality statistics in advertisements to attract patients (Wall Street Journal, July 28, 1987). Consumer groups believe they have won the day. They are delighted to have mortality data made available; these data give purchasers much needed information about the quality of health care they are buying.

The home care industry should follow the recent example of the hospital industry and move without haste to identify the health outcomes of its service if it does not want to be in the defensive position hospitals are in today. If the industry does not assume leadership in quantifying its health outcomes, the purchasers will inevitably define them for home care. Most likely the defined outcomes will be negative quasi-measures such as mortality data, and admissions to an institution.

If, however, the industry moves now to quantify positive health outcomes it will soon have the beginning of a national data base that describes positive, actual health status outcomes. And in one year, individual agencies will have positive health-outcome data to use internally and externally. Internally, client outcomes could be used to form the centerpiece of a strong quality assurance mechanism, and externally, client outcomes would give an agency a solid, quantifiable product to market to purchasers of home care services.

A meta-analysis of published and unpublished literature that addresses the concept of home care outcomes follows. After describing the current "state of the art", an approach to developing and measuring home care outcomes is posited.

A SELECTED REVIEW OF THE LITERATURE

In 1976, Januska presented the results of a national survey of quality assurance efforts in public health nursing. The major findings were a need for a diversity of methods and outcome standards. Then in 1979, Flynn and Ray surveyed the literature and the practice field, and noted "an interesting difference, since the Januska survey, is that agencies are increasing their efforts to develop outcome measures." However, Flynn and Ray also noted that many community health quality assurance programs were not accessible through the literature and that agencies often duplicated efforts.

The public status (i.e., published) of quality assurance efforts in community health is not much different today than in 1979, although some progress has been made in the quantity of research published (Werley & Fitzpatrick, 1984). In reviewing "quality of care studies" in 1984, Lang and Clinton concluded by advocating for more descriptive and comparative research designs and greater rigor in data analysis. Similarly in examining public health nursing research in 1984, Highriter noted a lack of consistency in the definition of "client outcomes", questionable methodology, weak designs, and a shortage of replication of studies.

Currently there is a bountiful supply of literature that addresses quality assurance and patient-outcome standards in general. This particular discussion, however, is offered not as a definitive review of all the theoretical and operational issues surrounding the concept of patient outcomes standards, but rather as a selected examination that focuses only on outcome standards in home care. The review addresses published, unpublished, and privately (not accessible through professional literature indexes) published documents. Its purpose is to stimulate thought, discussion, and action. By examining a variety of approaches to developing patient outcomes in home care, the major issues can be brought into focus. Furthermore, future practice and research directions can be thoughtfully decided upon from an informed perspective.

Approaches

The printed materials on outcome standards for home care come from a variety of perspectives. Although a possible categorization of perspectives would be to use the "education-practice-research" paradigm, the following more distinct categories will be used in this discussion: 1) generic outcome literature; 2) promulgated standards; 3) operational outcome standards; 4) program evaluation standards; and 5) standards derived from research. These are not mutually exclusive or exhaustive categories; however, this classification provides a useful framework for the purpose of this review.

Generic Literature

The generic literature documents the "why" and "how to" of developing outcome measures. Donabedian's 1976 "structure-process-outcome" framework is similar to the generic literature and has been integrated into nursing's quality assurance paradigm (ANA, 1976a). The reason for outcome measures is undisputed, yet Donabedian's explanation is worth repeating: "Health outcomes have an integrative property. . . . At the level of the individual patient, outcomes represent the result of the efforts of all those who have been involved in the patient's care. At the population level, health outcomes represent the operation of the health services system as a whole . . . ."

- 4 -

In the generic literature, two decade-old nursing publications remain relevant. The first is the American Nurses' Association's (ANA) Issues in Evaluation Research (1976b). This anthology provides a broad overview of the theoretical and methodological issues integral to research on outcomes. Furthermore, the text includes descriptions of the first two nursing research efforts to develop empirically valid patient outcomes (Horn & Swain, 1976; Hegvary, Gortner, & Haussman, 1976).

The second oft-cited reference is ANA's Guidelines for Review of Nursing Care at the Local Level (1976a). This guide offers a systematic model for developing outcome standards and provides the first contemporary published example of an outcome standard for home care (see Figure 1). Building on the ANA Guidelines and other sources, in 1980 the Minnesota Department of Public Health published specific instructions on how to develop outcome criteria for a variety of public health nursing services, including home care. However, the only example of an outcome standard offered in the Minnesota Department of Health publication is for a well child.

FIGURE 1

CRITERIA DEVELOPMENT WORKSHEET

TARGET POPULATION: Chronic Illness: Essential Hypertension

Variables   a. 35-50 years old
               b. Ambulatory
               c. Newly diagnosed or referred

Criteria Subset	Screening Criteria	Critical Time	Standard	Exception
Acts to minimize applicable risk factors	The patient will: Lose weight until ideal weight is attained	6 weeks – 6 months	100%	Obesity due to another disease
	Stop smoking	6 weeks – 6 months	100%	
Attains/maintains optimal physio-logical functioning	Have BP of no more than 160/96 when lying	6 weeks – 6 months	100%	
Knowledge of medication regime	Correctly identify medications by sight	6 weeks – 6 months	100%	Blind, retarded
Understands disease process	Explain in his own words: Nature of disease process	0 – 6 weeks	100%	
Assumes responsibility for own care	Measure own BP accurately	6 weeks – 6 months	100%	
Active involvement of significant others in therapeutic program	The significant other will: Verbalize knowledge of the therapeutic program	6 weeks – 6 months	100%	Patient with no significant others

(American Nurses' Association, 1976, Guidelines for Review of Nursing Care at the Local Level, Kansas City, MO: ANA, 1976, pp. 47-50.)

Promulgated Standards

Promulgated standards are those that are formulated by a group of experts and published by an organization. They are set forth by a recognized body; however, their usefulness, reliability, and validity may never be tested. Meeting a set of promulgated standards is voluntary; they tend to be general and may serve as a guide for developing more specific patient outcome standards. In home care, two types of organizations dominate standard setting: national professional groups and state associations.

Nationally, the National League for Nursing (NLN) (1987) has provided the only standards for all types of home care and community health agencies since 1966. The majority of these standards are structure- and process-oriented; however, since 1980 the NLN has required, for accreditation, that an agency demonstrate that it has met the following standards:

"12.1   Each [service] program has written objectives stated in measurable client-outcome terms." (NLN, 1987, p. 20)

"17.1   Annual program evaluation includes assessment of:
. . . . client outcomes." (NLN, 1987, p. 29)

The impact of these standards -- requiring client outcome measures -- will be discussed in the next section, Operational Outcome Standards.

The American Public Health Association (APHA) (1985) has published model standards for a variety of preventive health services including chronic disease control, communicable disease control, home health services, and mental health. The APHA standards include process and outcome "objectives"; Figure 2 provides an example of such an outcome objective.

The ANA (1987) publishes a wide variety of standards addressing clinical practice areas. Some of them are written as practice standards and include structure, process, and outcome standards for each component of practice (ANA 1982, 1986a, b). Figure 3 demonstrates that not all of the outcome standards are necessarily client-oriented. Other ANA (1983, 1985) standards are organized by nursing diagnoses and include client-oriented outcomes, as seen in Figure 4.

The second group of organizations which promulgate standards are state home health agency associations. These voluntary groups are patterned on the trade association model; however, there is an active "quality assurance" component within most of these groups.

In contrast to most promulgated standards, detailed outcome criteria based on medical diagnoses have been developed in Florida (Florida Association of Home Health Agencies, 1980) and Colorado (Colorado Association of Home Health Agencies, 1983), as seen in Figures 5 and 6, respectively. Although medically defined, both groups use nursing oriented domains to identify the subsets of criteria (note left-hand columns of Figures 5 and 6).

The Florida Association of Home Health Agencies also developed outcome criteria specific to physical therapy (1980a), speech pathology (1980b), and occupational therapy (1983) services. Although the basic format for the therapy outcomes is identical to that of the "skilled" nursing outcomes, not surprisingly, the criteria subsets vary slightly: both physical and occupational therapy add a "functional" subset, whereas speech replaces "physical" with criteria subsets specific to speech "impairments."

Assuming a different approach, Pennsylvania (Pennsylvania Association of Home Health Agencies, 1986) and Minnesota (Minnesota Assembly of Home Health

Nursing Agencies, 1985) have developed organizationally oriented standards which emphasize structure and process standards. Nonetheless, Pennsylvania's standards specify:

"Service Outcome: . . . The provider shall demonstrate that

. . . . Records indicate that projected outcomes were

accurate in at least 60% of the cases." (PAHHA, 1986)

The Minnesota standard similarly includes: "There shall be a care plan written for each client record. It will define client centered goals and objectives . . . ; (and) a provider shall perform record review to determine service outcomes on discharged cases . . . this review shall include . . . measuring change in functional level of client." (MAHHNA, 1985)

The Michigan Assembly of Home Health Agencies (1986) recently issued client outcome standards in response to productivity and cost control forces. In a position statement released by the Clinical Services Committee, the Michigan group specified: "Although quality is difficult to define, certain outcomes indicate whether quality services have been provided.

These outcomes include:

1.   The patient/family is knowledgeable of and participates in their
     health care plan of treatment.

2.   There is an improvement in the ability of the patient/caregiver to
     perform the patient's activities of daily living.

3.   Plan for alternatives has been established for care if #2 is not met
     . . . ." (MAHHA, 1986).

FIGURE 2

Goal: A full range of preventive, therapeutic and
long-term home health services will be delivered
within the community so that appropriate home
care services are available and utilized as a
responsible, feasible and desired alternative
to institutionalization. Residents of the
community with illnesses or handicaps which
restrict self-care but do not require acute
care or continuous supervision will be able
to continue living at home rather than in a
health care institution for as long as
desirable and feasible.

AREA: Home Health
       Services

FOCUS	OBJECTIVE	INDICATORS
	Outcome	
	O-1 By 19 ___ ___ percent of persons known to be in need of non-institutional supportive services will receive the appropriate level of services.	Percent of persons in need of services who receive them.
	O-1 By 19 ___ the percent of inappropriate placements in long-term care institutions will not exceed ___.	Percent of inappropriate placements.
Acute Care	P-4 By 19 ___ ___ percent of persons convalescing from specified surgical procedures, medical events and/or medical interventions will convalesce in the home with needed patient monitoring, dressing changes, and other necessary services provided in the home.	Hospital and home health agency records.
	Cross Reference: Institutional Services	
Availability and Access- ibility of .Services	P-7 By 19 ___ home care services necessary to meet client and family needs will be available and accessible to all those in need.	a. Volume of service and profile of clients served compared to demographic profile of community.
	7a By 19 ___ nursing and selected other home health services will be available, at least on an emergency basis, 24 hours a day, seven days a week, including holidays.	b. Presence of mechanisms to assure availability and access to those unable to pay.

(Exerpted from American Public Health Association, Model Standards: A Guide

for Community Preventive Health Services, 2nd ed., Washington DC: American

Public Health Association, 1985 pp. 41 and 77)

FIGURE 3

Standard VI. Intervention

The nurse, guided by the care plan intervenes to provide comfort, to restore, improve, and promote health, to prevent complications and sequalae of illness, and to effect rehabilitation.

.
.
.

Outcome Criteria

1. The client and family demonstrate self care to the extent of their ability.

2. There is measurable evidence of progress toward goal achievement.

3. The client and family use community resources appropriately.

4. Problems, interventions, and responses of the client and family are recorded in a systematic, retrievable, and timely manner.

5. There is documented evidence that interdisciplinary services are in accord with client needs and capabilities.

(Excerpted from Standards of Home Health Nursing Practice, Kansas City, MO: American Nurses' Association, 1986, pp. 11-12)

FIGURE 4

Outcome Standard IV. Self-Care Deficit

.

.

.

Criteria

The individual:

1. identifies factors that interfere with the ability to perform self-care
    activities.

2. identifies alternative methods for meeting self-care needs.

3. utilizes alternative methods for meeting self-care needs.

(Adapted from Outcome Standards for Rheumatology Nursing Practice, Kansas City,
        MO: American Nurses' Association, 1983, p. 6)

DIAGNOSTIC CATEGORY: CONSCIOUSNESS AND CONDITION

Specific Nursing Diagnosis	Process Criteria	Outcome Criteria
Total health management deficit: irreversible.	The nurse	The individual's hygiene, nutrition and elimination needs are met.
		The individual sustains no complications of immobility.

(Excerpted from Neuroscience Nursing Practice, Process and Outcome Criteria for
Selected Diagnoses, Kansas City, MO: American Nurses' Association, 1985, p. 9)

FIGURE 5

FLORIDA ASSOCIATION OF HOME HEALTH AGENCIES

OUTCOME CRITERIA

Target Population   Decubitus Ulcer
Service: Skilled Nursing

Criteria Subset	Outcome Criteria	Standards	Exceptions
Physical	1) Temperature is within 96 to 99	100%	Physician aware
	2) Healed ulcer No broken skin areas No redness, swelling No drainage Absence of pain	100%	
	3) Oral intake of 1500-2000 cc/ daily with output of clear amber urine	100%	
Safety	4) No evidence of hazards . . .	100%	
Psycho-Social	6) Patient and/or significant other demonstrates acceptance of condition by....	100%	Patient unwilling to discuss....
Education	7) Describes preventive measures:	100%	

(Adapted from Florida Association of Home Health Agencies Presents a Quality

Assurance Program, 2nd ed., Orlando, FL: Florida Association of Home Health

Agencies, 1980, pp. 47-48)

- 13 -

FIGURE 6

COLORADO QUALITY AUDIT FOR INDIVIDUAL CASE RECORD

Topic: Wound/Decubitis
Goal: Curing of disease process

Nrsg. Process Paramtr.	Outcome/ Goal	Assessment Parameters	Outcome Measurement Criteria	...	Abnormal Outcome Protocol
Physio-logical Assessment	Healed Wounds	S: Pain/dis- comfort	None		Document
		O: BP T P R	90-160/60-90 96.4-99 F (po) 60-90, reg. 16-20 at rest		Report to physician and team
		Ulcer site appearance Drainage	 None		Review treatment
		.	.		.
		.	.		.
		.	.		.
Psycho-social/ Environ-mental	Acceptance of treat-ment . .	Coping ability . . .	Verbalizes under-standing . . .		Seek consul-tation
Evalua-tion of compliance with Edu-cation & Treatment	Medication	Medication Intake/ Understanding	Teaching & verbalized understanding recorded		
Preven-tion of compli-cations	Absence of compli-cations	Chronic pain . . .	Asymptomatic . . .		Reassess in depth . .

(Excerpted from Colorado Quality Assurance Audit Criteria, Englewood, CO:
Colorado Association of Home Health Agencies, 1983, #13)

Operational Outcome Standards

Operational outcome standards are those that are actually in use in the practice field. None of the operational standards discussed here have documented reliability and validity measures; however, the fact that service agencies have made the standards operational strongly suggests face and content validity.

Like promulgated standards, these operational standards reflect a diversity of perspectives. They range from having programmatic (aggregate) to individual client foci, and address outcomes from a medical, nursing, and/or functional problem identification perspective.

Programmatic Standards

The Oklahoma Indian Health Service (IHS) is a multi-service community provider serving a large geographic area. Following the NLN's promulgated standard regarding program objectives, Oklahoma has developed aggregate client-oriented outcome standards based on medical diagnosis categories, as seen in Figure 7 (Oklahoma Area Community Health Nursing Program, 1986). A Louisiana home health agency has also developed programmatic standards as Figure 8 demonstrates (Steedley, 1979). Note however in the Louisiana example that although the "Program Objectives" are grounded in medical diagnoses (i.e., "acute illness . . . infective and parasitic diseases . . .), the outcome "indicators" are functionally defined (e.g., maximum rehabilitation). In contrast, the Visiting Nurse Association (VNA) of Metropolitan Atlanta's (1984) programmatic objectives, are consistently based on functional status as seen in Figure 9. Thus, although both the Oklahoma IHS's and the VNA of

Atlanta's program objectives were written from the NLN definition and although both agencies wrote aggregate standards, the health problems were defined from different perspectives: medical versus functional. It is also interesting to note that the Pennsylvania (1986) promulgated standards, and the operational Oklahoma (1986) and VNA of Atlanta (1984) standards all use 60% as a standard for goal achievement. Although there are other examples of programmatic outcome objectives based on functional status (Morris, 1979), the above examples adequately represent the file of available multidisciplinary program outcome objectives.

As noted earlier, Florida (1980, 1983) offers rehabilitation outcome standards for therapy services for individual patients based on medical diagnosis. In contrast, Figure 10 provides an example of social work programmatic objectives based on social work "health problems" (Visiting Nurse Association of Dallas, 1984). Thus, although some agencies address the issue of program objectives from a multidisciplinary perspective, it is also possible to isolate program objectives by the provider's discipline.

FIGURE 7

OKLAHOMA AREA COMMUNITY HEALTH NURSING PROGRAM

EMPHASIS PLAN

Outcome Objectives

1. By 1990 the number of identified diabetics under adequate long-term control defined as a blood sugar of less than 150 mg. for at least two years will increase by 5% annually.

2. By 1990, 60% of all identified hypertensives will be under long-term adequate control as defined by BP of less than 140/90 for at least two years.

3. By 1990 the prevalence of significant obesity defined as 120% of desired weight will be reduced 20% for all age groups without nutritional impairment.

(Excerpted from Oklahoma Area Community Health Service, Health

Promotion and Disease Prevention Emphasis Plan

as submitted in NLN Self-Study

June 1986, p. 12 h)

FIGURE 8

DATA UTILIZATION - FOR SUCCESSFUL
PLANNING AND EVALUATION
(HOME HEALTH SERVICES OF LOUISIANA, INC., NEW ORLEANS)

Agency goal translated into program objectives

Goal: To provide high quality comprehensive health care service through a
coordinated plan of treatement to the chronically ill, aged, and
disabled residents of the community.

Program Objectives

A. Given a three-month admission period to the program, at least 50% of
patients with acute illness will recover their health and demonstrate
actions which promote optimum health.

    INDICATORS

    Discharge category of "Maximum Rehabilitation" was indicative of
    patients recovering their health.

    Patients with primary admission diagnosis in the following categories
    were grouped into Acute Illnesses:

    1.   Infective and parasitic diseases;
    2.   Neoplasms with surgical procedures but without metastases;

    DATA SOURCE: A 10% random sample of charts ....

B. Given a four-month admission period to the program, at least 45% of
patients with chronic illnesses will achieve maximum recovery within
the defined limits of their diseases or disabilities.

C. At least 50% of patients in the terminal stage of their illnesses
and/or their families will demonstrate the ability to cope with the
emotional and physical aspects of a terminal disease.

(Adapted from M. L. Steedley, Data Utilization - For Successful
Planning and Evaluation, in Community Health: Today and Tomorrow,
NLN 1979, pp. 65-77, #52-1768)

FIGURE 9

VISITING NURSE ASSOCIATION OF METROPOLITAN ATLANTA

PROGRAM OBJECTIVES

Home Health Services

Overall Objectives

To assist those in need of therapeutic treatment services to regain functioning, to become rehabilitated to the extent possible, and to achieve stability of their pathological condition.

To assist those with chronic illness and disability to remain in their homes as long as it is safe, comfortable, and medically and functionally feasible for them to do so.

Supporting Objectives

1. To improve the functioning status of 70% of the patients who were in need of therapeutic treatment and admitted for home health services.

2. To assist 70% of the patients who on admission have an expected outcome of "independent" in functioning status to become independent at time of discharge.

3. Within two months of admission either to discharge or reduce service requirements of 55% of the patients admitted.

4. To achieve 60% of the goals established for patients.

(As quoted in Administrator's Handbook, New York: National League for Nursing, 1984, p. 108)

FIGURE 10

THE VISITING NURSE ASSOCIATION OF DALLAS

MSW Standards and Outcomes for Clients

Health problem diagnosis	Projected client outcomes	Acceptable client outcomes
1. Coping abilities, impairment of		
a. Inability to identify stress factors	1. Client/family verbally acknowledge state when in stress	1. 85%
	2. Client/family able to state cause of stress	2. 50%
b. Inability to identify options for relief of stress situation	1. Client/family behaviorally acknowledge the existing stress situation	1. 85%
	2. Client/family verbally acknowledge the stress situation	2. 70%

(Excerpted from MSW Standards and Outcomes for Clients, as reprinted in

Administrator's Handbook, New York: National League for Nursing, 1984, p. 360)

Individual Standards

Moving from the aggregate to the individual measures, operational standards continue to span the spectrum of medical, nursing, and functional perspectives.

As mentioned earlier, the Minnesota Department of Public Health (1980) published guidelines for developing outcome standards. The impact of the statewide effort is reflected in the operational standards created by agencies in Minnesota. The Minneapolis Department of Health (1984) developed individual client outcome criteria using the state guidelines (Decker, Stevens, Vancini, & Wedeking, 1979); however, the variance from the state promulgated model to the local operational standards is noteworthy. The state model is based on a medical diagnosis and the subsets address standards such as physical health, activities of daily living (ADL), diet, and medications, as seen in Figure 11. On the local operational level, both the City of Minneapolis (Minneapolis Department of Health, 1984) and the Ramsey County (Minnesota) Public Health Nursing Service (1981) used the medical diagnosis for problem identification as suggested by the state model. The subsets however, address knowledge of the problem and healing process, performance of the treatment, and lifestyle adjustments, as seen in Figure 12. Figure 12 also includes the subset of the physical status of the patient, a dimension not addressed in the Minneapolis Department of Health's standards. (Otherwise the two agencies use essentially the same standards).

Another statewide effort was reported in the literature by the Georgia Department of Human Resources (Kline, Tracy, & Davis, 1986); however, the outcome statements are global (e.g., "optimal total health . . .") and actually only the process standards are measurable.

Other agencies have developed patient outcome standards derived from a nursing diagnosis framework. Gould and Wargo (1985) have developed nursing care plans using nursing diagnoses and outcomes as the framework for documenting home care provided by nurses. As seen in Figure 13, the standards address the dimensions of patient knowledge and performance. Inver and Aspinall (1981) describe another method for developing performance-oriented outcome standards based on the "goal attainment scaling" method, as demonstrated in Figure 14. Although Inver and Aspinall's method was developed for inpatient use, the model is suggestive for home health.

One of the most well reported efforts for developing operational patient classification and outcome schemes is that of the federally funded Omaha VNA projects which commenced in 1976 (Simmons, 1980; Martin, 1982; Martin & Sheet, 1985; Simmons, 1986). Revising the expected outcome-outcome criteria schemes was a major focus of the most recent Omaha project and specific work on outcome standards will not be available until some time in 1987 (Personal Communication, 1986). The results of this most recent study will yield outcome scales (possibly similar to those described in Inver and Aspinall above) that address the dimensions of knowledge, behavior, and physical status.

One of the most specific and well conceptualized operational outcome schemes was developed by the VNA of Metropolitan Detroit (1984). The Detroit model is based on the Third Annual Conference on Nursing Diagnosis. The outcome schema is derived from the Karnofsky Performance Status Scale and Leavell and Clark's three "levels of prevention." Thus, like the Louisiana example (Figure 8), the Detroit VNA standards move from a nursing diagnosis problem to a functional status outcome as seen in Figure 15. The Detroit model uses a 3 x 3 framework for outcomes in which one of three severity levels is chosen, and within that level outcomes are defined for three dimensions: knowledge, performance, and physical status (Boucher, 1984). Although the Gould and Wargo (1985) and Detroit (1984) models both use a nursing diagnosis, the Detroit model more clearly distinguishes levels of severity and the various dimensions of client outcomes.

Finally, there is another group of operational standards that uses functional status for both problem identification and patient outcome. A multidisciplinary inpatient rehabilitation instrument, the LORS-II, (Posavec & Carey, 1982) is offered in Figure 16 because it is suggestive for home health. Both the LORS-II scale and the Inver goal attainment scale were developed for inpatient use and focus on the physical dimension although they can be used in home health. In contrast, the operational standards home health agencies use tend to be multidimensional, addressing knowledge as well as performance and physical status. Another difference between the inpatient and home care standards is the object of the standard: inpatient standards address the patient/client only, whereas home health standards tend to address the patient/client and the family/significant other, as seen in Figures 10, 11, 12, and 15.

Ramsey County (1986), in addition to the medical diagnosis specific outcomes, also uses an "ADL Function" assessment tool as seen in Figure 17. This tool is completed when the client is admitted to home care services and then again when the case is closed. By rating the client's functional status on a three-level independent-dependent scale for six ADLs, the client is assigned to one of fourteen categories of functional status. Theoretically this instrument allows quantification of the change in a client's functional status from admission to, and discharge from, home care services.

- 23 -

Visiting Nurse and Home Care, Inc. (1983) of Hartford-Waterbury (Connecticut) has developed a multidimensional outcome instrument as demonstrated in Figure 18. This Self-Management Outcome Criteria (SMOC) tool documents a client's level of independence on a four-point scale for each of five dimensions: knowledge, health promotion behavior, functional status, psycho-social status, and support status. The SMOC is completed on admission for actual and expected level of functioning, at 60-day intervals, and upon discharge. The SMOC tool is used in conjunction with more specific outcome criteria for physical status and other areas; however, the SMOC tool also theoretically allows quantifiable change measurement in functional status during the course of home care service delivery.

FIGURE 11

MINNESOTA DEPARTMENT OF HEALTH

OFFICE OF COMMUNITY HEALTH SERVICES

SAMPLE CRITERIA SET

TOPIC: Congestive heart failure
POPULATION: Adult in his own home
POINT IN TIME: Discharge from home health program

1. Cardiovascular status maintains stable pattern
    a.   Pulse rate between 60-90/min.
    b.   Respiratory rate 15-24/min-easy
    c.   Long sounds clear

2. Working toward maximum activity and ADL level
    a.   Plans rest periods

3. Patient and/or significant other has knowledge of and eats prescribed diet.
    a.   Prepares menus following prescribed diet.

4. Patient and/or significant other understands and follows medication
    regimen.

(Adapted from Decker, F., Steven, S. L., Vancini, M., & Wedeking, L.,
Using Patient Outcomes to Evaluate Community Health Nursing, Nursing Outlook,
April 1979 Vol. 27, #4, pp. 278-282.)

FIGURE 12

RAMSEY COUNTY PUBLIC HEALTH NURSING SERVICE

Client Outcome Criteria

Open Wound Requiring Dressing Change

1. Client and/or significant other understands healing process and its effects.
   (a) Client and/or significant other describes cause of wound
   (b) Client and/or significant other describes healing process of wound and/or complications of healing
   (c) Client and/or significant other relates healing process to own wound and prognosis of healing

2. Client and/or significant other understands management of healing process.

3. Client and/or significant other implements a management program, independently as able.

4. Client accepts necessary life style adjustment.

5. Client wound status
   (a) Redness, discharge, swelling or foul odor not present
   (b) Pain and tenderness in wound decreased
   (c) Depth and diameter of wound decreased

(Excerpted from Client Outcome Criteria, RCPHNS Record, Minneapolis, MN: Ramsey County Public Health Nursing Service, 1981)

FIGURE 13

UNITED HOME HEALTH SERVICES
PHILADELPHIA, PENNSYLVANIA

<u>Nursing Diagnosis:</u> Actual or potential impairment of skin integrity related
to: _____

Goal: Patient/significant other will be able to carry out those activities
necessary to restore and maintain skin integrity.

<u>NURSING ORDERS</u>

1. Assess general condition of skin: cleanliness, turgor, dryness,
temperature.

2. If breakdown is present, assess the following.....

3. ...

Contributing Objectives	Dates Instructed	Goal/Accom.
Patient/S.O. Will:		
Describe and maintain regime to keep skin clean and dry		
Demonstrate correct cleansing and/or dressing of ulcer (if applicable)		
Describe/demonstrate daily regime of inspection and massage of pressure areas		
Identify signs and symptoms of beginning decubitis		
Describe and implement a turning and movement schedule ...		
Keep lower extremities elevated (if applicable)		
Be familiar with the use of devices to relieve pressure ...		
Identify/eat foods high in protein, vitamins, iron		

Key - I = instruction - E = evaluation - N = narrative - C = care given ....

(Excerpted from Gould, E. J., & Wargo J.,
Home Health Nursing Care Plans.
Published by United Medical Services Inc., 1985,
5308 Rising Sun Avenue, Philadelphia, PA 19120
pp. 42-43 Kathleen Mauter)

FIGURE 14

Using Goal Attainment Scaling (GAS) Method

Example: Goal: To care for colostomy without assistance

Four components: remove soiled bag - irrigate - cleanse stoma - apply new bag

Step 1	Step 2	Step 3	Step 4	Step 5
Does none of above without assistance	Does 1 of above without assistance	Does 2 of above without assistance	Does 3 of above without assistance	Does 4 of above without assistance

(Adapted from Inver, F. & Aspinall, M. J.,
Evaluating Patient Outcomes <u>Nursing Outlook,</u> <u>29</u> (3), pp. 178-181)

FIGURE 15

VISITING NURSE ASSOCIATION OF METROPOLITAN DETROIT

NURSING DIAGNOSIS AND MANAGEMENT PROTOCOLS

Impairment in Skin Integrity Related to _____

I.   DEFINING CHARACTERISTICS

                                          Nursing Observations

       Disruption of skin surfaces   Monitor vital signs
       Destruction of skin layers   Response to treatment program
                                          . . . . .

II.   NURSING INTERVENTIONS
       Nursing Interventions   Health Teaching
       Nursing Treatments   Explain causes of impaired
       Reduce or remove   skin integrity
         causes of impaired   Rationale and intended
         skin integrity   effect of treatment program
       . . . .

EXPECTED OUTCOME STATEMENTS/NURSING ACTION CUES

Level I	Level II	Level III
A. Patient demonstrates knowledge related to impaired skin integrity in ____ visits 1. Signs/symptoms 2. Influencing factors 3. Sequence/complications	A. Patient/caregiver demonstrates knowledge related to impaired skin integrity within _____ visits.	A. Patient/caregiver identifies/demonstrates knowledge related to severe impairment in skin integrity within ____ visits. 1. Signs/symptoms . . . . .
B. Patient identifies/demonstrates measures to prevent/correct impaired skin integrity within _____ visits.	B. Patient/caregiver identifies/demonstrates measures to control/correct impaired skin integrity within ____ visits.....	B. Patient/caregiver identifies/demonstrates measures to manage severe impairment in skin integrity within _____ visits .....

Level I	Level II	Level III
C. Patient achieves/main- tains skin integrity within _____ weeks.....	C. Patient exhibits control of impaired skin integrity within _____ weeks	C.Patient exhibits healing/ control of severe impairment in skin integrity within _____ weeks.....

(Excerpted from Guide for the Development of the Nursing Care Plan, Detroit, MI: Visiting Nurse Association of Metropolitan Detroit, 1984)

FIGURE 16

LEVEL OF FUNCTION SCALE (LORS-11)

RATINGS (completed on admission, discharge follow-up)

Activities of Daily Living

Rated by:

		RN	OT	Ranges 0 to 4

A. Dressing
B. Grooming
C. Washing/bathing
D. Toileting
E. Feeding

0 = Pt. does not perform the function
4 = Pt. performs the function reliably and independently

Mobility
(Check and rate one)

			RN	OT
Ambulation (if poss.)	1.			
Wheelchair management	2.			

Communication

Verbal   RN   ST

A. Auditory comp.
B. Oral expression

Gestural

Written
A. Reading comp.
B. Written expression

(Adapted from Posavec, E. J., & Carey, R. G.,
Using a Level of Function Scale (LORS-II)
to Evaluate the Success of Inpatient
Rehabilitation Programs, Rehabilitation Nursing
7 (6), pp. 17-19)

FIGURE 17

RAMSEY COUNTY PUBLIC HEALTH NURSING SERVICE

ADL Function Code

	A	B	C
Bathing			
Dressing			
Toileting			
Transferring			
Continence			
Feeding			

Indepen-dence   Depen-dence

	A	B	C

Indepen-dence   Depen-dence

Open   Close

8. Independent in feeding, continence, transferring, toileting, dressing, and bathing.

6c. Dependent in bathing and one additional function both of which are at the C level.

2B. Dependent in all six functions of which 3 or more are at the B level.

(There are 14 different categories in all)

(Excerpted from RCPHNS 1986 Agency Form)

FIGURE 18

VISITING NURSE AND HOME CARE, INC.
(Hartford & Waterbury, Connecticut)

SELF MANAGEMENT OUTCOME CRITERIA

Areas	High 0	1	2	Low 3
1. Level of knowledge	Describes/ demonstrates accurate application of knowledge/ skills	States knowledge/demonstrates skills with reinforcement/guidance/ supervision	Ready to learn but has -limited/inaccurate knowledge -difficulty with articulation/ application -lack of confidence	Unable or unwilling to learn or apply knowledge Lack of readiness (denies, disagrees with, or does not recognize need)
2. Reduction of risks to health	Minimizes risks associated	Minimizes risks/ complies with reinforcement	Risk avoidance/ compliance vacillates.....	Unable or unwilling to minimize risks .....
3. Functional ability/ ADL management	Self manages personal care, household duties, and.....	Self manages but with difficulty	Manages with assistance only	Unable or unwilling to manage
4. Behaviormentation emotion	Social behavior appropriate	Aware of and compensates for behavioral or mental.....	Awareness and/or compensation vacillates	Unaware of deviations .....
5. Support from significant other(s)	Receives needed support from s.o.(s)	Receives needed support from s.o.(s) and community agencies.....	Receives needed support from community agencies only	Unable or unwilling to use available support.....

(Excerpted from Visiting Nurse and Home Care, Inc., Rev. 1983, 146 New Britain Ave., Plainville, CT 06062)

Program Evaluation Standards

Another source of outcome standards is program evaluation research literature. In an effort to document the impact of home care services, these studies define outcomes from the researcher's perspective, usually concentrating on economic, physical, or functional measures.

Fagin (1982) offers a review of the economic impact of nursing interventions. Many of these studies address community-based interventions, in order to demonstrate dollar savings by preventing institutionalization. Economic outcomes, although significant, are not equitable with patient outcomes. Once reliable and valid patient oucomes are established, the financial worth of home care services may be better documented.

Maternal-child health studies provide a popular opportunity to document the impact of home visits. Barkauskas (1983) defined outcomes for mothers and infants using the dimensions of physical status, behavior, and satisfaction. Barkauskas's population was essentially healthy, although at risk; however, the findings yielded no significant differences between visited and not-visited mother-infant pairs.

In another study however, addressing a population of very low birth-weight infants, the authors concluded that "early discharge . . . with follow-up care in the home by a nurse-specialist, is safe and cost-effective" (Brouton, et al, 1986). Outcome measures in this 18-month study included rehospitaliza- tions, acute care visits, and standard measures of physical and mental growth. Outcomes for mothers and infants delivered by lay midwives were examined in another study (Sullivan & Beeman, 1983). Maternal outcomes of this study included: length of labor, blood loss, medical care requirements, and hospital admissions; infant outcomes included: birth weight, Apgar score, medical care requirements, hospital admissions, and mortality.

The VNA of Metropolitan Atlanta used less rigorous methodology to define the outcomes of cancer patients receiving home care services from them. They were: functional status, hospitalization, and reason for discharge (recovered, stabilized, deceased, hospitalized, and nursing home admission) (Legge & Reilly, 1980). In the Cleveland VNA, the outcomes for mental health patients were defined as hospital readmission, employment status, social behavior, and compliance with medication regimen (Vincent & Price, 1977).

A number of studies have looked at the outcomes of elderly clients who receive a broad range of community-based social and health services. The On lok demonstration (Ansak & Zawadski, 1984) identified the following outcome measures: health, functional (ADL) and cognitive status, institutionalization, and service costs. In another California study (Miller, Clark, and Clark, 1985), a similar evaluation of a different type of community-based care initiative, the Multipurpose Senior Services Project, identified outcomes as longevity, nursing home days, and hospital days. Although client data in terms of ADLs, Instrumental ADLs (IADL), and mental status were collected, the program evaluation did not address these outcomes. However, in the Triage study (Quinn & Hodgson, 1984), ADL, IADL, and mental status variables, as well as cost and institutionalization outcomes, were all defined and measured as outcomes.

Finally, in a retrospective record study of a geriatric home care, program outcomes were defined in terms of client discharge status: to self or informal care, to an institution, to formal community-based care, or death (Day, 1984).

The program evaluation studies tend to focus on the more objective and reliable outcome measure of whether or not a client is admitted to a hospital or nursing home. This proxy outcome measure was not addressed in any of the promulgated or operational outcome standards. The studies reviewed in this section suggest that outcome standards for "acute" home care services may not be serviceable for "chronic" populations. Or, it may be that operational standards (as defined in this paper) are difficult to translate into reliable research variables. Certainly more than one researcher has called into question the reliability of the patient care record as a source of valid information (Koerner, 1981; Day, 1984; Baldwin & Lueckenotte, 1986).

Related Research

The issues of reliability and validity plague the quest for useful outcome standards. Intraprofessionally, the nursing profession has been confounded by the development of nursing diagnoses (Hurley, 1986). Kim (1986) and others (McLount, 1986; McLane, 1986) suggest that nursing must clinically validate nursing diagnoses prior to testing interventions and developing outcomes.

More pragmatic scholars recall Donabedian's (1976) delineation of two different causality issues in relation to outcomes: 1) establishing causal validity between process and outcome standards from a quality assurance perspective (i.e., has the available scientific knowledge been properly applied?); and 2) establishing clinical validity (i.e., does the clinical procedure cause the intended outcome?). Lang and Clinton (1984) suggested that the nursing profession acknowledge this difference and leave the clinical questions to the clinical scientists while allowing the quality assurance professionals to pursue Donabedian's first issue.

If one steps back into the mid-1970s, two efforts to establish patient outcomes empirically stand out: the Rush-Medicus System (Hegvary, Gortner, & Haussman, 1976) and the Horn and Swain Measures (1977). The Rush-Medicus system addresses three dimensions of patient outcomes: physical condition, psychological status, and health knowledge, and is organized around nursing process parameters. The Horn-Swain study yielded 348 reliable and valid outcome measures organized in a 9 x 4 matrix: nine health dimensions derived from Orem's self-care theory (air, water, food, elimination, rest/sleep, solitude/social interaction, protection, normality, and health deviation) and four domains within each dimension: physical status, knowledge, skills, and motivation. Both of these tools were developed with adult inpatient populations. Although the literature does not suggest either instrument has been tested in the community, the similarity of the subsets of standards (physical status, knowledge, behavior, etc.) to those of the operational standards discussed earlier suggest some of the inpatient work might be testable in the home care field.

Currently the Home Care Association of Washington (HCAW), under a federal grant, is developing and testing outcome scales for home care. The first three scales -- General Symptom Distress, Discharge Status, and Taking Prescribed Medicines have been developed and tested for reliability and validity. HCAW's quality assurance manual (Lalonde, 1986) describes the purpose, completion, reliability, and validity of each scale along with how to use them for quality assurance. The author notes ". . . standards for the outcomes presented in this manual have not yet been set . . . at the moment standard setting is up to the discretion of each home care agency. Although much work is needed to link the process of home care service delivery with these outcomes, the scales provide the opportunity for generating outcome standards for populations of home care patients.

Other literature suggest nontraditional methods and variables to be addressed in evaluating home care outcomes. Harris (1981) advocates using client satisfaction and multisource interviewing to measure at least one dimension of client outcomes in home care satisfaction. Padilla and Grant (1985) and Ferrans and Powers (1985) suggest quality of life as a valid outcome and are working on instruments to measure this multidimensional concept.

THE DIMENSIONS OF THE CONCEPT

From the prior discussion and examples, it is clear that a <u>health outcome</u> <u>is a measurable change in client's state of health related to the receipt of</u> <u>health care services</u>. Thus to define a health outcome, one must examine the concepts of change, client, health, the relation between health care and health, and health care services. The complexity and variety of outcome statements described in this paper reflect the inherent multiplicity of definitions of these concepts used to characterize "outcomes." To understand outcome better, it will be useful to consider briefly each of the terms used in its definition.

CHANGE: Although there is general agreement that a change is an objective, observable, and measurable phenomena, some authors have advocated measuring change through interviews and self-report, using subjective and nonobservable data. However, as the quantitative-qualitative dichotomy is resolved, it appears scientists will opt to use both types of measures in defining change. Thus, change is probably one of the simpler concepts in the definition of outcomes.

CLIENT: In the tradition of public health, home care providers identify the client as an individual, family, target group, or community. This discussion does not address examples of family-oriented or community-oriented outcome standards, although they exist. Nonetheless, it appears that the intersection of the client as an individual and the client as the family (or significant other) is the unique target of home care providers. Even when an aggregate is the focus of the program objective (goal statement for a group), the object continues to be the elusive client/family phenomenon.

HEALTH: Health can be defined from a number of perspectives. In the inpatient setting, it may be easier to define it than in the community. The preceding discussion suggests defining health from a medical, nursing, or functional perspective; or from an "acute" versus "chronic" health problem perspective. However, by viewing nursing's domains to include all five dimensions (physical, behavioral, psychosocial, knowledge, and functional well-being), it is possible to resolve the conflict between the medical-nursing-functional trichotomy and the acute-chronic dichotomy (see Figure 19).

RELATION: As discussed earlier, this causal link involves two distinct questions: one for the applied, quality assurance, professional; and one for the pure, clinical scientist. Quality assurance professionals must focus on the current available knowledge and strive to demonstrate the process-outcome link between health care and health. The questions of scientific causal relations between treatment and health status must be left to clinical researchers.

HEALTH CARE SERVICES: Home care providers represent a myriad of professional disciplines, paraprofessional services, and informal caregivers. For the process-outcome links to be established, the sources and interaction effects among these services will eventually have to be examined.

This discussion yields a matrix of potentials for defining "outcomes" as seen in Figure 20.

Given that the vast majority of home care is provided by the Registered Nurse (RN), Home Health Aid (HHA), and Informal Caregiver, nurse researchers may want to focus on the illustrated subsection of the cube (Figure 21).

Those to whom the advancement of nursing knowledge is a priority will direct their inquiries across the outcome spectrum focusing on the top layer of the cube (diagonally striped area). However, public policy demands require a different emphasis in focus: How do home care services impact physical and functional dimensions of health? (vertically striped areas). Although there is overlapping in terms of the knowledge sought, the foci of inquiry are different. If nurse researchers fail to assume leadership in answering the public policy questions posed at the ends of the outcome spectrum, others will; and in doing so they will, albeit inadvertently, define significant portions of nursing's practice domain.

FIGURE 19

DIMENSIONS OF HEALTH

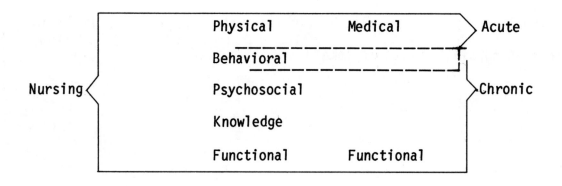

FIGURE 20

MATRIX OF POTENTIALS FOR DEFINING "OUTCOMES"

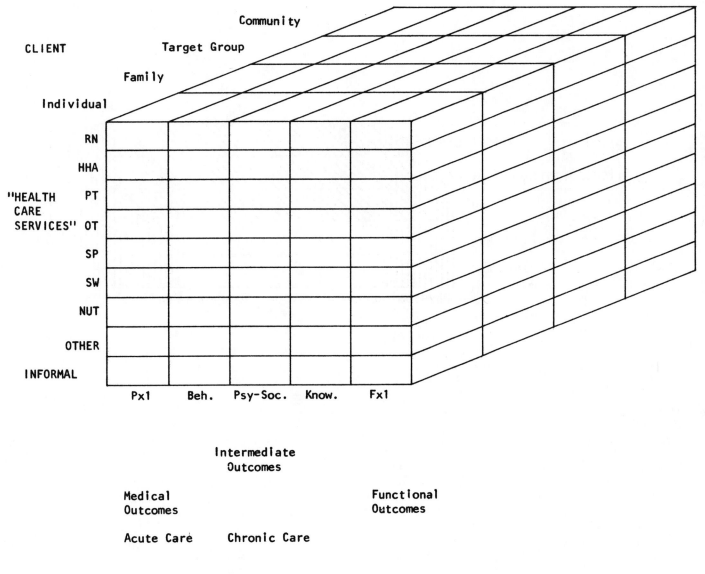

FIGURE 21

SUBSECTION OF "OUTCOMES" MATRIX

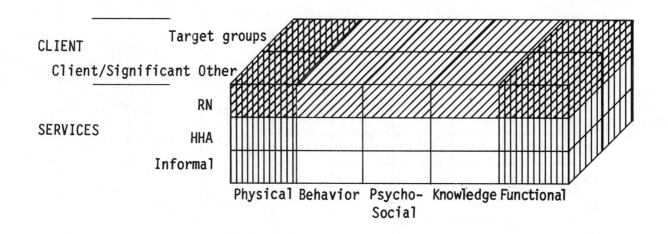

MOVING TOWARDS DEFINING HOME CARE OUTCOMES

This analysis suggests a framework that can be used to start to define and measure home care outcomes. The framework emerges from the works reviewed here and the need to develop aggregate-level outcome statements which can be applied in service delivery setting and be measured by empirically valid methods. The approach is based on the idea of "client-oriented program objectives" as suggested by NLN's Criteria and Standards (1987).

Client Outcome Program Objectives

Client outcome program objectives (COPOs) are measurable, client-oriented goal statements, written for a particular population that is served by a specific health program. These goal statements describe the intended results of care rather than its process; they are descriptions of client behaviors and/or health status that will be demonstrated upon discharge from a health service program. A well-written client outcome program objective consists of four components describing:

1) Who is to demonstrate the outcome;

2) What the outcome is;

3) When the outcome is to be demonstrated; and

4) How many will demonstrate the outcome.

For example, a home care agency strives to improve the functional independence of the clients it serves. This is a broad goal, applicable to a traditional Medicare home care program. However, it might also be the goal of a specialized rehabilitation home care program. Translating this general goal into a client-oriented program objective might result in the following statement: "70% of all clients admitted with ADL deficits will be discharged with an improved level of independent functioning within three months of service."

Who: All clients admitted with ADL deficits.

What: Improved level of independent functioning.

When: Within three months of service.

How many: 70%

Now the questions are "what is an ADL deficit" and "what is an improved level of independent function"? These are relevant issues, and one of the primary concerns an agency needs to address early on in the process of developing COPOs is: What can we measure? If an agency has an ADL measurement tool that is completed on initial assessment and at the time of discharge, the above example will be an easy COPO to make operational.

The issue of what data the agency can collect needs to be considered throughout the process of developing COPOs. Sophisticated specific objectives that cannot be evaluated are an academic exercise. It may well be that in the first years of this process, the agency's COPOs will be fairly general, limited by the agency's data collection resources. However, the ability to quantify some outcome indicators now will establish the framework for developing more specific positive outcome objectives in the future.

Developing COPOs

Given the above consideration regarding data collection resources, there are five steps to follow when developing COPOs:

1) Define the problem.

2) Define the outcome.

3) Define the population.

4) Define the numbers.

5) Design the evaluation mechanism.

1) Define the Problem

Health care services are provided to people with actual or potential health problems. How each agency defines its health problems that it treats may impact how the agency's COPOs are stated. Basically, health problems can be defined from at least three different perspectives: medical, nursing, and functional. In most cases, all three perspectives are used in home care: admitting a client based on a medical diagnosis, providing services based on a nursing care plan, and discharging a client based on functional status. There is no one "correct" perspective; however, for the sake of conceptual clarity, it is useful for each agency to identify how it characterizes its clients' health problems.

2) Define the Outcome

Defining the health problems an agency treats is a prelude to defining the outcomes of its service. The outcomes or goals of service can be viewed from

the same three perspectives as is done with the problem. Consider for example
the following:

Perspective	Problem statement	Outcome/Goal statement
Medical	Decubiti	Heal decubiti
Nursing	Interruption in skin integrity	Achieve and maintain skin integrity
Functional	Bedbound	ADLs with one person assist

Although a problem statement based on a perspective may suggest a
particular outcome statement, note that systematic COPOs do not require that
the problem statement dictates the form of the outcome statement. That is, an
agency may quite logically choose to define the health problems it treats from
a medical perspective and its outcomes or goals from a nursing and/or
functional perspective. A number of factors need to be considered in choosing
which perspective the agency wants to use in framing its COPOs, including the
agency's philosophy, program organization, documentation resources, and
reimbursement demands. Nonetheless, it is the author's bias that the
functional status perspective has particular merit in terms of defining
outcomes. The rationale for this bias is philosophical as well as practical.
Philosophically, home care is rooted in a tradition of teaching clients how to
independently maintain and promote their own health. Practically, functional
status categorizations (ADLs, IADLs, etc.) are understood across health care
disciplines and by consumers.

Putting aside the conceptual question of perspective, consider what actual
outcomes is expected that the clients achieve. Basically client outcomes for
home care services can be categorized as: acquisition of knowledge,

acquisition of skills needed to promote health, and improved health status.

For each service program, client outcomes in each of these three areas can be identified. For example, a traditional generalized home care program may expect the following types of outcomes:

Knowledge	- clients can correctly verbalize their medication schedule
	- clients can verbally identify signs and symptoms requiring a medical evaluation
Behavior	- clients can appropriately administer insulin
	- clients perform wound care
	- clients monitor blood pressure
Health Status	- wound heals
	- achieves complete rehabilitation, is independent in all ADLs
	- infection resolves

To start, an agency may want to choose the major health problems among the clients it serves and define program objectives for those clients. Or if it has already identified specific service programs (e.g., oncology, rehabilitation, pediatrics, chronic care), the agency can identify one or two major outcomes for the clients of each of those services. An agency may want to choose outcomes that are realistic and measurable. If for example the agency serves a large diabetic population, the medical or health status goal of controlling the diabetes is probably not realistic or very easily measured, especially during the course of service. However a behavioral outcome regarding the client's ability to physically manage his or her diabetic care (insulin administration, urine testing, diet preparation, etc.) is realistic. Often, the most realistic outcome for an agency to project for problems around medication administration is that clients have the knowledge they need to manage their medications. If, however, the caseload includes many clients with wounds, wound healing or the absence of infections may be appropriate outcomes for the service program. Furthermore, for a hospice program death at home may be the major outcome desired.

The goals or outcomes can take many forms. The keys to identifying which goals to incorporate into COPOs are:

a)   Is it a client outcome, either in terms of knowledge, behavior, or physical health status?

b)   Is it significant to the overall mission?

c)   Is it measurable given the data collection resources available?

3) Define the Population

Once major outcomes have been identified, who will achieve those outcomes needs to be defined. Again, data collection resources need to be considered during the process of defining the population. If clients are admitted to the agency and then assigned an identification number that also reflects admission to a specific service program (e.g., hospice, oncology, pediatrics, etc.), then it is feasible to define populations by service program. If, however, the client identification scheme does not discriminate by service program, but the COPOs identify populations by service program, then evaluation will require manual retrieval (e.g., chart reviews) of the data.

Defining populations is best illustrated by considering some examples. A common goal is "clients know (can verbalize) their medication schedule." That is simple enough and an agency might expect that all its clients are discharged with this knowledge. But what about those who cannot grasp this knowledge, such as children, incapacitated older people, or the mentally impaired? There are at least two approaches to resolve this: 1) define the population as "adult clients" and then when the percentage is defined or how many, consider the fact that not all adult clients can be expected to achieve this outcome; or 2) define the population as "all clients and/or their caregivers." The fact is that in home care an individual client is rarely serviced; the target of service often includes family, significant others, or the generic "caregiver."

In some cases the population targeted for the outcome will not include the client at all. For example, with a hospice program, although one COPO may be "clients die at home", another COPO may be "family or caregiver(s) manage (have the knowledge and psychomotor skills) pain control regimen." Another case is chronic ventilator dependent children; one COPO may be "parent manage equipment maintenance."

Let us consider another common outcome -- wound healing. There are wounds that are expected to heal and there are others that are chronic in nature and the best that can be expected is that the client (and/or caregiver) will master wound care skills. It may be that for an early discharge, post-surgical program, basically all the clients are expected to achieve wound health (the anticipated exceptions can be dealt with when defining "how many"). Whereas in a generalized home care program, an agency may want to redefine the population of clients with wounds into two groups: 1) those with chronic wounds, and 2) those with temporary wounds.

One final example is the outcome of "improved functional independence." This outcome is fairly general and will apply to a majority of an agency's caseload. However, a standardized measurement tool is needed (which can be as simple as rating clients on a three-point scale -- independent, partially independent, dependent -- on the basic six ADLs) and some population parameters. The target population will probably not include children (development gains are more appropriate outcomes than functional independence), and will exclude the severely and chronically dependent. If the ADL tool can be translated into numeric scores, the population may be defined as "adult clients with an ADL score of 3 to 5." If the tool is not quantifiable, the population may be defined as "adult clients with partial dependence in one or more ADLs."

Again, defining the target populations for specific outcomes will be dependent on the agency's data retrieval resources. An agency may define one or two major outcomes for each service program and define the population as all the clients admitted to the program. This is a realistic and logical approach. The expected failures (clients who won't achieve the outcome) can be accounted for when the "how many" of the COPO is defined.

4) Define the Numbers

Now there is an outcome (the "what") and a target population (the "who") -- two of the four components of a COPO. The remaining components are numeric: a) "when" the client is to achieve the outcome; and b) "how many" clients are expected to realize the outcome.

The "when" is usually fairly simple. If the agency's average length of stay with a client is two months, then a "when" of three months is probably safe. Greater specificity can be achieved if an agency has length-of-stay data by medical diagnosis, nursing diagnosis, functional status, and/or service program. (Medical diagnosis is known to be a poor predictor of home care need; nonetheless, if the COPOs are framed from this perspective, length-of-stay information based on medical diagnosis will be useful data for projecting this component of the COPO.)

Usually calendar time (days, weeks, month) is used to define the time frame for a program objective. However, an agency may want to consider using the number of home visits or the number of hours of service in defining this component of the COPO. The rationale for calendar time is twofold: a) it is more general and allows for variances in client need in terms of the number of visits required by an individual to achieve a certain outcome; and b) calendar time is more readily understood by purchasers of health care than the number of visits. (From a consumer perspective, contrast these statements: "You will learn how to manage your diabetic care at home within two months" vs. "You will learn to manage your diabetic are at home within twelve visits.")

Finally, the other consideration in defining "when" is "how many." The two numbers have a direct correlation, as described below.

The "how many" is usually a percentage of the defined population. For example, "80% of all adult clients admitted to the hospice program" or "70% of all adults admitted with partial ADL deficits." The first rule is that this percent is never defined as "100%." This is in contrast to process standards where "100%" is a commonly used threshold. It is realistic to expect a plan of care to be documented for 100% of the clients; the agency has sufficient control over this type of process to establish a standard of 100%. However, in home care, an agency never has enough control to assure 100% realization of particular client outcome.

Establishing a realistic standard for "how many" requires a data base or an informed, experienced guess. In the initial year of developing and using COPOs, an agency may choose to develop a data base on which to project a percentage figure. In such a case, in year one of using COPO's the "how many" may be addressed by general references such as "increase" or "decrease." For example, in year one the COPO may read: "Increase the number of adult clients able to correctly verbalize their medication schedule within one month of service." The next step is to design a way to find out what percent of adult clients realize this outcome within one month; for example, 60% achieve the outcome within the stated time frame. (Yes, there are issues of documentation involved and that is how COPOs operate within a quality assurance program.) In year two, the COPO can be developed as: "70% of all adult clients are able to correctly verbalize their medication schedule within one month of service." As the quality of the agency's service and documentation improves this figure can be reviewed upward. However, at some point below 100%, a realistic maximum will be achieved. (Note: This example describes a client outcome achieved "within one month of service", not necessarily an outcome demonstrated at the time of discharge. In general COPOs will address discharge outcomes, however for this particular outcome it makes sense, in practice, to expect it is achieved prior to discharge. The point is COPOs must be grounded in practice if they are to be realistic and useful for promoting quality.)

The other approach to defining "how many" is based on experience. Given an agency's caseload, the defined outcomes, and defined populations, what is the best guess at how many clients will achieve the outcome? Many will feel comfortable projecting that "70% of all clients admitted with newly diagnosed insulin-dependent diabetes will be able to independently manage their care at home within three months of service." Basing the standard (the percentage) on informed clinical judgment is a rational approach to defining this component of the COPO. It also provides the agency with a measurable goal against which to evaluate the effectiveness of its services at the end of year one. The home care outcome literature is not sufficiently mature to provide any useful resource around establishing this statistic. The most commonly cited statistic is 60% or 70% in terms of achieving particular outcomes in home care. These figures show up in promulgated standards (standards developed by an expert group, not standards developed from actual clinical practice) and are probably a reflection of the adage "a third get better with your help, a third will get better without your help, and the other third will never get better." Nonetheless, either approach in year one of using COPOs is acceptable: use "increase" and/or "decrease" and develop a data base, or use a percentage based on clinical experience.

Finally, as mentioned above, this standard of "how many" needs to be balanced with the "when" figure. In general, the higher the percent, the longer the time frame for achievement will be, and vice versa. For example, consider the COPO stated above: "70% of all clients admitted with newly diagnosed insulin-dependent diabetes will be able to independently manage their care at home within three months of service." If an agency's data base allows it to determine that the average length of stay for a client with this diagnosis is two months, and that 90% of these clients are discharged to self-care at home, then the abovestated COPO is probably realistic. Yet the agency might decide to decrease the time frame to two months from three months, and likewise will want to decrease the percent expected to achieve the outcome. Now the COPO will be: "60% of all clients admitted with newly diagnosed insulin-dependent diabetes will be able to independently manage their care at home within two months of service."

A minor digression here -- the above COPO is an example of defining the population from a medical perspective and defining the outcome from a nursing and functional perspective. The assumption is that the agency has a protocol defining "managing diabetic care at home independently." That protocol will be reflected in the individualized client outcomes in the client's plan of care. Another approach to this particular COPO is to define the outcome from a medical perspective, that is: "60% of all clients admitted with newly diagnosed insulin dependent diabetes will have a stable blood glucose of 100 mg/dl to 200 mg/dl within two months of service." In this latter example, to evaluate the objective, the agency will need to have a mechanism to measure blood glucose levels for each client. As mentioned earlier, the medical outcome may be narrow and difficult to evaluate. In this case one has to assume that a stable blood sugar reflects the client's ability to independently manage his or her care at home.

5) Design the Evaluation Mechanism

Although this is the final step in the formal process of developing COPOs; it is also a step which has been considered throughout the process -- what are the agency's data collection capabilities? If this question has been thought about throughout the process of defining the problems, goals, populations, and numbers, this step is very easy.

Each COPO is technically the statement defining the four components of who, what, when, and how many. To make the COPO operational a fifth component is needed -- the evaluation mechanism which needs to be designed specifically for each COPO.

As this mechanism will vary with each agency's data collection capabilities, a couple of examples can be considered here. Once the COPO is developed, the evaluation mechanism will naturally evolve from the COPO statement itself. Consider this COPO: "70% of all adult clients will be able to correctly verbalize their medication schedule within one month of service." Evaluation may be achieved any number of ways, the only guideline is that the evaluation mechanism be defined up front and introduced with the COPO. Methods to evaluate the above COPO include: 1) 100% of client records are manually reviewed at discharge for evidence that the objective was met in the time frame established; 2) all client records reviewed at quarterly utilization review meetings are evaluated for evidence of meeting this objective; or 3) medication teaching and client knowledge evaluation are documented via a computerized system, and a monthly summary of clients who achieve this objective is generated by the system. Any of the above three evaluation mechanism can be employed, the question is "What is a realistic evaluation plan given your agency's resources?"

Another example is: "70% of all adult clients admitted with an ADL score of 3 or less are discharged with an improved level of independent functioning within three months of service." The evaluation mechanism may be: 1)a manual review of all client records at discharge; 2) a manual review of all, or a random sample of all, client records of clients admitted with an ADL score of 3 or less; or 3) ADL scores are entered into the computer system at admission and discharge and a monthly summary of discharges is generated that identifies how many clients achieved the outcome within the time frame stated.

These two examples provide an idea of different approaches to evaluation. At this time, given that home care outcomes are in the infancy of their development, sophisticated evaluation mechanisms are not necessary. The major point is that the evaluation mechanism is realistic for an agency to manage.

Summary

Client-oriented program objectives (COPOs) provide a structure to evaluate the quality of an agency's services and to demonstrate accountability to the consumers of its services. Agencies are encouraged to take a proactive stance and to examine their major service programs in light of the client outcomes their home care services are intended to achieve. Development of one or two major COPOs for each service program can be easily managed using the steps outlined in this article.

References

American Nurses' Association (1976a). Guidelines for review of nursing care at the local level. Kansas City, MO: American Nurses' Association.

American Nurses Association (1976b). Issues in evaluation research. Kansas City, MO: American Nurses' Association.

American Nurses' Association (1982). Standards of psychiatric and mental health nursing practice. Kansas City, MO: American Nurses' Association.

American Nurses' Association (1983). Outcome standards for rheumatology nursing practice. Kansas City, MO: American Nurses' Association.

American Nurses' Association (1985). Neuroscience nursing practice, process and outcome criteria for selected diagnosis. Kansas City, MO: American Nurses' Association.

American Nurses' Association (1986a). Standards of community health nursing practice. Kansas City, MO: American Nurses' Association.

American Nurses' Association (1986b). Standards of home health nursing practice. Kansas City, MO: American Nurses' Association..

American Nurses' Association (1987). ANA Publications. Kansas City, MO: American Nurses' Association.

American Public Health Association (1985). A guide for community preventitive health services (2nd ed.). Washington, DC: American Public Health Association.

Ansak, M., & Zawadski, R. T. (1984) On lok CCODA: a consolidated model. In Community-Based Systems of Long Term Care. Philadelphia: Haworth Press, 147-169.

Baldwin, K. A., & Lueckenotte, A. G. (1986). Use of nursing diagnosis in community health agencies using the PORS. In M. E. Hurley (Ed.), Classification of Nursing Diagnosis: Proceedings of the Sixth Conference. St. Louis, MO: C. V. Mosby, 330-337.

Barkauskas, V. H. (1983). Effectiveness of public health home visits to primaparous mothers and their infants. American Journal of Public Health, 73 (5), 573-580.

Brouton, D. et al. (1986). A randomized clinical trial of early hospital discharge and home follow-up of very-low-birth-weight infants. New England Journal of Medicine, 15, 934-939.

Colorado Association of Home Health Agencies (1983). Colorado quality assurance audit criteria. Englewood, CO: Colorado Association of Home Health Agencies.

Day, S. R. (1984). Measuring utilization and impact of home care services: A systems model approach for cost-effectiveness. Home Health Care Services Quarterly, 5 (2), 5-24.

Decker, F., Stevens, L., Vancini, M., & Wedeking, L. (1979). Using patient outcomes to evaluate community health nursing. Nursing Outlook, 27, (4), 278-282.

Donabedian, A. (1976). Some basic issues in evaluating the quality of health care. In American Nurses' Association Issues in Evaluation Research. Kansas City, MO: American Nurses' Association, 3-28.

Fagin, C. (1982, June). The economic value of nursing research. Presented at Council of Nurse Researchers meeting, Biennial Convention of American Nurses' Assocation, Washington, DC.

Ferrans, C. E., & Power, M. J. (1985). Quality of life index: development and psychonetic properties. Advances in Nursing Science, 8(1), 15-24.

Florida Association of Home Health Agencies (1980). Presents a Quality Assurance Program (2nd ed.). Orlando, FL: Florida Association of Home Health Agencies, 85-138.

Florida Association of Home Health Agencies (1983). Presents a quality assurance program (2nd ed.): Occupational therapy addendum. Orlando, FL: Florida Association of Home Health Agencies.

Flynn, B. C., & Ray, D. W. (1979). Quality assurance in community health nursing, Nursing Outlook, 24 (10), 651-653.

Gould, E. J., & Wargo, J. (1985). Home Health Nursing Care Plans. Philadelphia: United Medical Services, Inc., 42-43.

Harris, M. D., 1981. Evaluating home care? Compare viewpoints. Nursing & Health Care, 2 (4), 207-209, 213.

Hegvary, S. T., Gortner, S. R., & Haussman, R.K.D. (1976). Development of criterion measures for quality of care: The Rush-Medicus experience. Issues for Evaluation Research. Kansas City, MO: American Nurses' Association, 106-114.

Hegvary, S. T., and Haussmann, R. K. D. (1976). Monitoring nursing care quality. Journal of Nursing Administration, 6 (9), 3-9, 12-16, 18-27.

Highriter, M. E. (1984). Public health nursing evaluation, education, and professional issues: 1977 to 1981. In Werley, H. H., & Fitzpatrick J. J. (Eds.), Annual Review of Nursing Research. New York: Springer, 165-189.

Horn, B. J., & Swain, M. A. (1976). An approach to development of criterion measures for quality patient care. In Issues for Evaluation Research. Kansas City, MO: American Nurses' Association, 74-82.

Horn, B. J., & Swain, M. A. (1977). Development of criterion measures of nursing care. Volumes I and II. Hyattsville, MD: National Center for Health Services Research.

Hurley, M. E. (Ed.) (1986). Classification of Nursing Diagnosis: Proceedings of the Sixth Conference. St Louis, MO: C. V. Mosby.

Inver, F., & Aspinall, M. J. (1981). Evaluating patient outcomes. Nursing Outlook, 29, (3), 178-181.

Januska, C., Engle, J., & Wood, J. (1976). Status of quality assurance in public health nursing. Presented at American Public Health Association Annual Meeting, Washington, D.C.

Kim, M. J. (1986). A Janus view, in Hurley, M.E. (Ed.), Classification of Nursing Diagnosis: Proceedings of the Sixth Conference. St. Louis, MO: C. V. Mosby, 1-14.

Kline, M. M., Tracy, M. L., & Davis, S. L. (1986). Quality assurance in public health. Nursing & Health Care, 1 (4), 192-196, 207.

Koerner, B. L. (1981) Selected correlates of job performance of community health nurses. Nursing Research, 30 (1), 43-48.

Lalonde, B. (1986). Quality Assurance Manual of the Home Care Association of Washington. Edmonds, Washington: Home Care Association of Washington, 38.

Lang, N. M., & Clinton, J. F. (1984). Assessment of quality of nursing care. In Werley, H. H., & Fitzpatrick, J. J. (Eds.), Annual Review of Nursing Research. New York: Springer, 135-163.

Legge, J. S., & Reilly, B. J. (1980). Assessing the outcomes of cancer patients in a home nursing program. Cancer Nursing, 3 (5), 357-363.

Martin, K. (1982). A classification system adaptable for computerization. Nursing Outlook, 30, (9), 515-517.

Martin, K., & Sheet N. (1985). The Omaha system: Implications for costing community health nursing. In Shaffer, F. A. (Ed.), Costing Out Nursing: Pricing Our product. New York: National League for Nursing, 197-206.

McLane, A. M. (1986). Summary and recommendations, in Hurley, M.E. (Ed.), Classification of Nursing Diagnosis: Proceedings of the Sixth Conference. St. Louis, MO: C. V. Mosby, 133-138.

McLount, A. (1986). Nursing diagnosis: Key to quality assurance. In M.E. Hurley (ed.), Classification of Nursing Diagnosis: Proceedings of the Sixth Conference. St. Louis, MO: C. V. Mosby, pp. 133-138.

Michigan Home Health Assembly (1986, November-December). Position Statement of Clinical Services Committee: Productivity expectation outlined by Michigan assembly. National Association for Home Care Newspaper.

Miller, L. S., Clark, M. L., & Clark, W. F. (1985). The comparative evaluation of California's multi-purpose senior services project. Home Health Care Services Quarterly, 6 (3), 49-79.

Minneapolis Department of Health (1984). In Fish, C., Administrator's Handbook, New York: National League for Nursing, 376-377.

Minnesota Assembly of Home Health Nursing Agencies (1985). Standards for home health care providers. Minneapolis, MN: Minnesota Assembly of Home Health Nursing Agencies, 15, 20.

Minnesota Department of Public Health (1980). Section of Public Health Nursing. Outcome auditing: One component of a quality assurance package. Minneapolis, MN: Minnesota Department of Public Health, 22.

Morris, H. H. (1979). A model for evaluating a community health agency. In Community Health: Today and Tomorrow. New York: National League for Nursing, 15-36.

National League for Nursing (1987). Accreditation Program for Home Care and Community Health: Criteria and Standards. New York: National League for Nursing.

Oklahoma Area Community Health Nursing Program (1986). NLN Self-Study. Oklahoma City, OK.

Padilla, G. V., & Grant, M. M. (1985). Quality of life as a cancer nursing outcome variable. Advances in Nursing Science, 8(1), 45-60.

Pennsylvania Association of Home Health Agencies (1986). Home health service provider standards. Harrisburg, PA: Pennsylvania Association of Home Health Agencies, 12.

Personal communication (December 1986) with S. S. Resner, Project Officer, Division of Nursing, Department of Health and Human Services.

Posavec, E. J., & Carey, R. G. (1982). Using a level of function scale (LORS-II) to evaluate the success of inpatient rehabilitation programs. Rehabilitation Nursing, 7 (6), 17-19.

Quinn, J. L., & Hodgson, J. H. (1984). Triage: A long term care study. In Community-Based Systems of Long Term Care. Philadelphia: The Haworth Press, 171-191.

Ramsey County Public Health Nursing Services (1981). RCPHNS Record. Minneapolis, MN.

Ramsey County Public Health Nursing Service (1986). ADL Function Codes. Minneapolis, MN.

Simmons, D. A. (1980). A classification scheme for client problems in community health nursing. Rockville, MD: NTIS Publication #HRA 80-16.

Simmons, D. A. (1986). Implementation of nursing diagnosis in a community health setting. In Hurley, M. E. (Ed.), Classification of Nursing Diagnosis: Proceedings of the Sixth Conference. St. Louis, MO: C. V. Mosby, 151-155.

Steedley, M. L. (1979). Data utilization - for successful planning and evaluation, in NLN Community health: Today and tomorrow. New York: National League for Nursing, 65-77.

Sullivan, P. A., and Beeman, R. (1983) Four years' experience with home birth by licensed midwives in Arizona. American Journal of Public Health, 73 (6), 641-645.

Vincent, P., and Price, J. R. (1977). Evaluation of a VNA mental health project. Nursing Research, 26 (5), 361-367.

Visiting Nurse and Home Care, Inc. (1983). Guidelines: Self-Management Outcome Criteria. Plainville, CN.

Visiting Nurse Association of Dallas (1984). In Fish, C., Administrator's Handbook. New York: National League for Nursing, 360.

Visiting Nurse Association of Metropolitan Atlanta (1984). In Fish, C., Administrator's Handbook. New York: National League for Nursing, 108.

Visiting Nurse Association of Metropolitan Detroit (1984). Guide for the Development of the Nursing Care Plan. Detroit, MI.

July 28, 1987. Wall Street Journal.

Werley, H. H., & Fitzpatrick, J. J. (Eds.). (1984). Annual Review of Nursing Research, Vol. 2. New York: Springer.

Simmons, R. P. (1980). Comprehensiveness in a nursing diagnosis. In Kim, M. J. & Moritz, D. A. (eds.), Classification of Nursing Diagnosis: Proceedings of the Third Conference. St. Louis, MO: Mosby, pp. 132-

Stumph, A. L. (1979). Data utilization for successful planning and evaluation. In NLN Community Health care: Today and tomorrow. New York: National League for Nursing, 55-62.

Sultz, H. A. and Young, K. (1997). Interview: Performance with home health care: Indexes in Arizona. American Journal of Public Health, 72(11), 127-88.

Thomas, F. and Pender, N. J. (1977). Evaluation of a WIN mental health. Nursing Research, 26, 151-207 SC.

Washington State Department of Health. (1984). Self-sufficiency. Olympia: State of Washington.

United Nations Association of the United States. (1982). Administrator's Handbook. New York: National League for Nursing, 20.

Washington Nurse Federation of Professional Affairs. (1982). In First City Washington's Handbook. New York: National League for Nursing, 62.

United Nurse Association of Colorado. (1980). Nurse facts. Consider the interview of the Nursing Care Plan. Colorado Springs, CO: UNA.

Wall Street Journal.

Wilson, A. and Fitzgerald, R. (eds.). (1980). World Book of Nursing. St. Louis, MO: Mosby.